# GUIDE TO BREAST RECONSTRUCTION AFTER MASTECTOMY

## WHAT TO DO AFTER YOU ARE DIAGNOSED

### BEN J. CHILDERS, MD, FACS

Published by Ben J. Childers, M.D., F.A.C.S., Riverside, California.

The author and publisher have strived to be as accurate and complete as possible in the creation of this book.

This book is not intended for use as a source of medical advice. The information in this book is intended to provide basic information on breast reconstruction procedures and the subjects discussed. It is not intended to be comprehensive by any means. The book is not intended to diagnose or to treat any medical conditions, or to replace the advice of the reader's physician(s).

The reader should regularly consult a physician in matters related to his or her health, specifically with respect to any symptoms that may require diagnosis or medical attention. For diagnosis or treatment of any medical problems, consult your physician(s).

The author and publisher are not responsible or liable for any damages or negative consequences from any treatment, action, application or preparation to any person reading or following the information in this book.

While all attempts have been made to verify information provided in this publication, the author and publisher assume no responsibility for errors, omissions or contrary interpretation of the subject matter herein. Any perceived slights of specific persons or organizations are unintentional.

Any trademarks mentioned in this book are listed for reference purposes only and are the property of the respective trademark owners.

# Table of Contents

# Note From A Patient

*I was referred to Dr. Childers following a series of failed reconstructive surgeries and a rather complex right breast mastectomy with extensive scarring. Before meeting with Dr. Childers, I consulted with four reputable plastic surgeons, which refused to operate on me due to the complexity of my case.*

*Dr. Childers accepted the challenge with confidence, gave me hope, patiently listened and addressed my questions and concerns, educated me on the plan and the steps involved, and assured me that the reconstruction could be done.*

*The reconstruction journey took over a year, and was complicated and hindered by an unexpected lumpectomy, slow healing, and my not so cooperative skin. Dr. Childers was always there for me. He was always compassionate, caring, professional and patient. He is knowledgeable and experienced, and he carefully and flawlessly performed every procedure. As a result, he created a beautiful breast. My entire experience with Dr. Childers, from the first consultation, series of surgeries, to all follow up appointments, was very pleasant. He and his staff went above and beyond to make me feel cared for, warm and welcome.*

*Dr. Childers is a brilliant, gifted surgeon. He is certainly the best plastic surgeon I have ever encountered.*

*I am thrilled with the results, and I am back enjoying life again thanks to Dr. Childers.*

*Sincerely,*

*L. R.*

6

# Introduction

Ben J. Childers, M.D., F.A.C.S. is a Board Certified Plastic Surgeon, a Fellow of the American College of Surgeons, and a member of the American Society of Plastic Surgeons. He practices at and is the owner of Riverside Plastic Surgery Associates, Inc. in Riverside, California. He also owns Sheer Beauty Medical Skin Care boutiques in Upland and Redlands, California.

Dr. Childers earned his BA degree in Chemistry from Eastern Kentucky University, graduating Cum Laude. He received his Medical Degree at the University of Louisville Medical School and competed his internship in General Surgery at Beth Israel Hospital Harvard Medical School. He completed his residency in General Surgery at Beth Israel Harvard Medical School and his residency in Plastic Surgery at Loma Linda University. Dr. Childers also completed a fellowship in Hand and Microsurgery at Beth Israel Deaconess Medical Center at Harvard Medical School.

When women are diagnosed with breast cancer, many times they have a lot of stress and anxiety and don't know what to do. They often don't want to think about the future, but with good survival rates, they should consider the outlook for their long-term appearance.

In this book, Dr. Childers discusses some of the considerations for women who have been diagnosed with breast cancer and some of the first steps they should take after they are diagnosed. He provides an overview of options for breast reconstruction after mastectomy and he gives answers to some of the most common questions that patients will have. Dr. Childers also addresses a number of questions that patients have never considered asking, but should be asking.

# Questions And Answers

*When a woman is diagnosed with breast cancer, there is likely stress and anxiety. What are some of the first things she should do at that point?*

Typically when a woman has been diagnosed with breast cancer, she'll be called by the doctor to come in and go over some pathological results. There may be some tests that need to be done, but once she gets the diagnosis, then there are several things that go through her mind.

Much of the time patients will wonder if they're going to die. They may panic at first, but usually after they get over that, the surgeon describes the recommend treatments, whether it's going to be radiation or chemotherapy or surgery. The next thing that they usually think of is, "How am I going to look after the procedures that are planned?"

One of the first things a woman needs to do, after she gets the diagnosis, is go see a plastic surgeon, because the plastic surgeon can give a broad overview of what can be done to reestablish appearance after the mastectomy or other procedures. The plastic surgeon will work with the general surgeon and the radiation oncologist.
Depending on the patient's insurance plan, there may be a one-stop medical center where the patient is referred to all of the medical specialists. Usually, there's one person that coordinates consultations with the various specialists, but the plastic surgeon can give the patient a broad overview of alternatives for reconstruction. If not automatically referred to a

plastic surgeon, the patient should seek consultation with a plastic surgeon to make sure she understands the options related to her long-term appearance.

Although it is more common practice today for the general surgeon to refer the patient to a plastic surgeon before the mastectomy, there are still some surgeons that go ahead and perform the mastectomy without taking into account options that could make a breast reconstruction more successful for the patient. If dealing with an HMO, for instance, it is more likely to be automatically referred because that type of plan is comprehensive care.

I see a number of patients that come in and they are in tears because they've been diagnosed with cancer. They're going to lose their breast and they have no idea what they're going to look like. Once we get through with talking about some reconstruction options, they leave the office feeling much better about what's going to happen. Then they can go to their general surgeon and consider their options.

*In a general sense, what is meant by breast reconstruction?*

Breast reconstruction in its simplest sense is restoring the form of the breast. We're giving a patient her breast back. Reconstruction involves either reconstructing one breast and then matching it with the opposite breast or reconstructing both breasts to give natural form.

Function generally is difficult to restore. Once a patient has had a mastectomy, she's not going to be able to produce milk, because the nipple-areolar complex is gone. In some instances, the general surgeon may choose to spare the nipple-areolar complex. This is done on a case-by-case basis; however, milk production in that instance is not possible.

*What are some of the reasons a woman might want to consider breast reconstruction after she is either going to lose her breast or she already has?*

One of the main reasons is because they want to restore their feminine look and they want to feel a sense of wholeness, because a lot of women don't feel womanly without having their breasts. A lot of women, when they have mastectomies, have lost their self-esteem. They don't feel pretty; they feel like they've lost a part of their body. In many instances, when the reconstruction is done, they do feel that sense of wholeness, they feel that sense of femininity, and their self-esteem has gone back to where it was, and maybe even farther than it was before.

Another reason is in the fit of clothing. It's very hard sometimes, if a woman has had a mastectomy, to wear their clothes. Women's clothing is designed for a woman with a chest, so they feel uncomfortable that they have to pad. Women can get prosthesis, but the prosthesis has to be put in. Sometimes they get hot, they get sweaty, and so it's not as functional. They like to be able to get up in the morning, take a shower, put on their clothes, and have the breast that's there.

There are some women that really don't want reconstruction. Some women are okay with the mastectomy without reconstruction, but the vast majority of women do want some sort of reconstruction.

*Are there any other things that a patient should be considering when they're trying to decide whether or not to have the reconstructive surgery?*

Their personal life and work status is important to consider. Some procedures require more post-operative recovery than others. Some patients don't have the option of taking enough time off of work for reconstruction and recovery. They may need to pick an option where they can take a week off here and there. We've had some patients that had mastectomies and they came in two or three years later, when they could take the time off of work for the reconstruction and recovery.

Support from the family is obviously very important. There are women that have a very good support system where the husband or the mom, or dad even, is very supportive, and they do much better. Sometimes patients will seek psychological counseling when they have to go through this. They don't necessarily need to see a psychiatrist, but if they're depressed, then that needs to be treated.

*With the technologies available today, is it possible for a woman to regain her figure after a mastectomy and breast reconstruction?*

The answer is yes, with the clarifier that it's based on the figure or physique the patient is starting with. If we start with a figure that is easier to reconstruct, we can end up with a better result most of the time. For example a patient that is obese and weighs 300 or 400 pounds will be a lot more difficult to reconstruct than one who's 5'4" and weighs 130 pounds.

Sometimes we even enhance the figure from the perspective of the patient. We've had patients that had small breasts before the cancer and in the course of the reconstruction they decided they would like to have larger breasts, with a fuller look, and we were able to accomplish that during the reconstruction.

*Who are good candidates for breast reconstruction?*

Most patients that have breast cancer and will be having breast surgery are candidates for reconstructive surgery. Going to the plastic surgeon, upon initial diagnosis is a good place to start. The plastic surgeon can look at the type of cancer they have and will work with the oncologist to understand the treatment plan. By and large, most patients are candidates for reconstruction, but it needs to be discussed and the patient has to be evaluated to determine what type of reconstruction they can have.

*There was an indication that someone that was very obese would be difficult and that some patients don't want reconstruction. Are there any other indications that a patient would not be a good candidate for reconstruction?*

Depending upon the specific treatment protocol and how the body reacts to treatment can affect the ability to perform reconstruction with some methods. Sometimes, radiation treatment, and the amount of radiation, makes the breast tissue that's remaining very scarred and unyielding to the point where we are limited in the ability to perform certain reconstructive procedures.

Sometimes, the general surgeons will take out so much breast skin that there's not enough left to expand. Some of the general surgeons perform pretty aggressive mastectomies. Studies have shown the effectiveness of skin-sparing mastectomies, where a lot of the breast skin is spared. The areola and the nipple are removed, but all of the skin does not have to be taken. The skin of the breast doesn't have the cancer; it's the breast tissue itself. Now sometimes there are cases where the tumor will get close to the skin and the skin has to be taken. The skin-sparing mastectomy is something that's been around for many years now and it's something I would highly advocate for women to have.

*As a plastic surgeon, are there some options related to breast reconstruction where an initial consultation with you would affect the choice of the specific type of surgical treatment for breast cancer removal based on the patient's desire for a good appearance after breast cancer treatment?*

From the standpoint of treatment of the cancer, the patient's oncologist develops the treatment plan, based on the type and the extent of the cancer. By being involved before the surgery, a plastic surgeon can coordinate with the general surgeon to ensure that the tissue removal surgery is done in a manner that better accommodates the reconstruction, such as in conserving the skin or starting the reconstruction in combination with the mastectomy.

*If a patient has cancer in one breast are there some conditions that would indicate removal of the second breast?*

Lobular cancer is one of the cancers that we see, and it has a 20% occurrence rate on the opposite breast. Most patients who have been diagnosed pathologically with lobular cancer on one breast will undergo bilateral mastectomies.

*Is there a likelihood of a better cosmetic outcome if both breasts are removed and reconstructed?*

Women want two breasts that look the same with good symmetry. Regardless of the reconstruction procedures we use as plastic surgeons, there is a challenge in performing procedures where the two breasts look perfectly similar. Even with two natural breasts there is some lack of symmetry. One of the things I tell the patients is that your breasts are sisters, they're not twins. It may sound funny, but it's true. They are related, but they're not exact. What we try to do is to reconstruct them to where they can have as much symmetry as possible when they're wearing a dress or a bathing suit.

Sometimes, we can do a reconstruction on one side and then we have another breast that we have to do a reduction on, but those breasts don't necessarily look the same because on one side we're dealing with natural tissue and on the other side we're dealing with an implant that's round and spherical. When viewed, particularly without clothing, the natural breast on the opposite side may be saggy, and even if it has been lifted, is going to look different.

Many women in their younger years, in their 30s to 40s, that get cancer on one side, will choose to have bilateral mastectomies and then to have bilateral reconstruction to obtain the best possible symmetry.

Another point is that many women don't want to go through all of the surgery and reconstruction on one breast and then get cancer in the other breast five years down the road. The oncologist and the general surgeon give the patient the risks of future cancer development, but I've seen many that have had cancer, and then five or six years down the road they develop cancer in the opposite breast.

*We're also hearing about women that have a high cancer risk due to genetics and they chose to have both breasts removed due to the high risk. Was this the case with Angelina Jolie?*

There is a group of women that test positive for a mutation of the BRCA1 gene. Due to mutation, their genetics makes them much more susceptible to developing breast cancer later in life. Most of these women decide to undergo bilateral mastectomies prophylactically. For those women, we actually take off the breasts and then do immediate reconstruction. Angelina Jolie was one of these cases where she tested positive for the BRCA1 gene mutation and decided to have a double mastectomy and reconstruction. She did not have the cancer, but she had the mastectomies to prevent it. Her choice to perform double mastectomies decreased her chances of developing breast cancer from 87% to 5%.

This genetic testing is not routinely performed on all women; however, women with a history of breast cancer in their family should request that their physician or an oncologist perform the test. The thing about it is there are some people that don't want to have the test because they don't want to find out the answer. It's hard to believe, but that's the way humans are. They need to be prepared to do something when they get the answer. For those testing positive for the mutation, we would recommend bilateral mastectomy.

*If a patient makes a decision to have a prophylactic bilateral mastectomy plus reconstruction, would that all typically be done by a plastic surgeon?*

It can be and I actually prefer doing the mastectomy myself because it lets me be a little bit more cautious of the tissue. It allows me to do the mastectomy in a manner that best facilitates the reconstruction. This is not compromising any oncological aspect, because the goal here is to get rid of the breast tissue. It could be done either in collaboration with the general surgeon, or it could be done entirely by the plastic surgeon.

*There are cases where a patient chooses to defer any breast reconstruction due to time constraints, but typically if a patient has breast cancer and will be having a mastectomy and reconstruction, would the breast reconstruction typically be started or performed at the same time as the mastectomy?*

Yes, many times we perform the reconstruction at the time of mastectomy, depending on the pathology. It's prearranged with the plastic surgeon working with the general surgeon. It does depend upon the extent of the cancer and the results of a biopsy during the breast removal procedure. In the typical case, the patient has a breast cancer mass, the general surgeon performs the mastectomy, and they do a biopsy on the sentinel lymph node to ensure the cancer had not spread. If the sentinel node biopsy result is negative, usually we can go ahead and progress and do the initial reconstruction.

If that biopsy is positive, then they're going to need to have a lymphadenectomy, and that's setting the patient up for possibly needing radiation. We don't like to initiate the reconstruction at that time when there is a significant chance of radiation treatment. Many times we go ahead and plan for the reconstruction. We've got everything set, and then it's completely dependent on that sentinel node biopsy. If it's negative, then we'll go ahead and proceed on with the immediate reconstruction. If it's positive, then we'll just stop and wait until the radiation therapy is completed and perform the reconstruction at a later date.

*The treatment plan for some patients where the cancer mass is small, involves a combination of a lumpectomy and radiation treatment instead of full removal of the breast with a mastectomy. For such a patient would breast reconstruction still be considered?*

There are times when the result looks pretty good after the lumpectomy and radiation treatment. The breast still has a good shape, but yet it's a little smaller than the opposite side. The breast may need to be shaped a little bit, which can be done. Opposite side matching procedures, such as mastopexy, augmentation or reduction can be considered.

*Are breast implants always used for breast reconstruction or are there other alternatives?*

Either breast implants are used or alternatively we can use body tissue from the patient. There are patients that don't want an implant. They would like to use their own body tissue. That's possible in women who have some excess fat in the lower abdomen or back that we can use to reconstruct the breast. There has to be enough tissue that we can remove and still close the patient to be able to do that procedure.

*How are breast implants supported in a patient that has a mastectomy?*

Patients that have a skin-sparing mastectomies where the surgeon has been able to preserve a large amount of breast skin can have enough tissue to support the implants and the many times we can perform an immediate reconstruction. In early 2013, Angelina Jolie underwent three months of medical procedures, including double mastectomy and reconstruction. Skin-sparing techniques were used.

Other times we need to first implant a tissue expander that we put underneath the tissue. Usually it's underneath the pectoralis major muscle, where we expand the muscle along with expanding the skin. With this process, slowly over time in our office, fluid is placed within the tissue expander and it slowly stretches and gets larger and larger. This stretches the skin so that we can come back later, take out the tissue expander, and put in a permanent implant.

Sometimes tissue support is needed at the lower portion of the breast rather than just setting the breast implant under the skin after the mastectomy. There is a new method of tissue support being used called an acellular dermal matrix, or ADM. We may use this tissue to build a framework underneath the implant to support it. The use of ADM's is not without problems. Seroma (fluid accumulation) around implants, lack of incorporation of ADM into surrounding tissue, and infection, may complicate reconstruction. Please discuss the use of these products with your plastic surgeon.

*Are the implants used with breast reconstruction the same as the implants used for breast augmentation? Are there choices related to implant shape and type of material?*

The types of implants used for breast reconstruction are the same as the ones used for breast augmentation. For either procedure there are a number of choices to be made during consultation with the plastic surgeon. The choices relate to the material used in the implants, such as silicone or saline, the shape of the implants and size. There are three main breast implant brands, Mentor®, Natrelle® and Sientra®. Although there are some slight differences between these brands, I consider them to all have excellent products.

First, there are silicone implants and then there are saline implants. The silicone implant has a silicone shell with a cohesive silicone gel on the inside. This is commonly referred to as a "gummy bear" implant. If you cut the silicone implant with a knife, the implant actually stays together like a gummy bear, whereas the older silicone implants had a silicone shell and a silicone fluid on the inside.

Saline implants are similar to silicone implants. They have a similar silicone shell, but inside of the shell is a saline, or saltwater fluid. It's the same kind of water that we put in the veins when IV fluids are needed. The saline implant has a port or a valve where we put a little tube that is used to fill up the implant. They come in a variety of sizes and there is a maximum amount of saline solution that can be filled into them. The saline implant can rupture and, if they do, the saline fluid will leak into the body and the implant will deflate. Although such a ruptured implant will need to be replaced, the saline solution inside does not present a health risk if it leaks into the body. My own findings are that the saline implants tend to not last as long as the silicone implants.

One of the reasons that women will choose a silicone implants and why I would recommend them is that the silicone implant has a softer, more natural feel to it than the saline implant. The saline implant is going to be a bit firmer. The silicone is denser, so it tends to not wrinkle as much as the saline implant, and thus retains the shape better. I recommend that patients have their plastic surgeon show them both types of implants during their consultation, so they can feel the difference in softness.

More recently we have had anatomically shaped implants available in addition to the traditional round implants. Round implants give a fuller breast at the top while the shaped implants provide a more natural shape with fullness at the bottom of the breast. Choice between these types depends upon several factors. For breast augmentation procedures, the choice of implant shape is based on the way the patient's body is shaped and preference of the patient. When performing breast reconstruction on one side, we are trying to match the breast on the other side, so the choice is more determined by the shape that will best match the other side. If the patient is having a bilateral mastectomy, and thus the reconstruction will be done on both breasts, the patient's preferred breast shape and the expertise of the surgeon will determine which shape will be used.

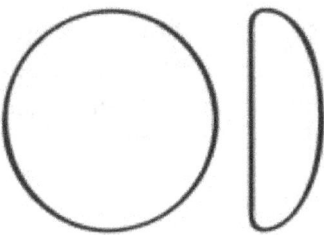

**Round Shape Implant**

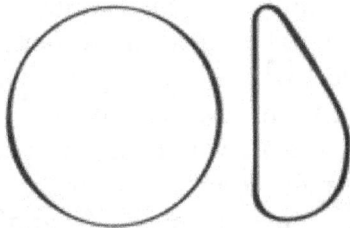

**Anatomical Shape Implant**

**Breast Implant Shapes**

In a similar manner, size of the implant used will depend on the type of procedure. If one breast is being reconstructed, then the best match to the opposite breast will determine the size of the implant. If both breasts are being reconstructed, then the patient generally will have choices of size as well as shape.

Size has been a limitation. The largest silicone implant is 800cc; however, larger silicone implants will be available in the near future.

Patients may also hear about textured and smooth implants, but the choice between these two types is really based on the surgeon's preference to achieve the best outcome and long-term results for the patient.

*How long will breast implants last? Do they need to be replaced after a certain amount of time?*

Recently, the implant companies warranty the implants for life, for either a manufacturing defect or for a malfunction where the implant ruptures. In my experience the implants generally will last 10 to 25 or 30 years. With the newer design implants, we don't really have complete longevity information other than the fact that the implant manufacturers are warrantying them for life. I usually tell patients that if it's not broken, it doesn't need to be fixed. There are ways to monitor the implants over time to check the integrity. With a saline implant, you can tell immediately when there's a leak because it just deflates rapidly. Mammography and MRI scans are very good at evaluating implant stability.

*Will reconstruction with breast implants preclude being able to detect cancer in the future?*

Having the implants doesn't really preclude being able to detect cancer. The mainstays of breast cancer detection after mastectomy is doing a monthly breast examination, feeling the breast, making sure that nothing has changed. There is the possibility of breast cancer recurrence in the skin. Women might see a mass in the skin or a change in the skin, so they need to be looking at their skin that's left and they also need to be feeling their breast to have a good baseline feel of what their normal breast feels like. If anything changes from that, then they need to visit their doctor. I would also recommend seeing your plastic surgeon once yearly.

*What are some of the alternative reconstruction procedures where the patient's tissue is used for reconstruction instead of implants?*

When we take a patient's tissue from one part of the body to use for reconstructing the breast we refer to the section of tissue as a flap. The breast is primarily fatty tissue and in this type of reconstruction we are moving a flap of fatty tissue to replace fatty tissue in the breast.

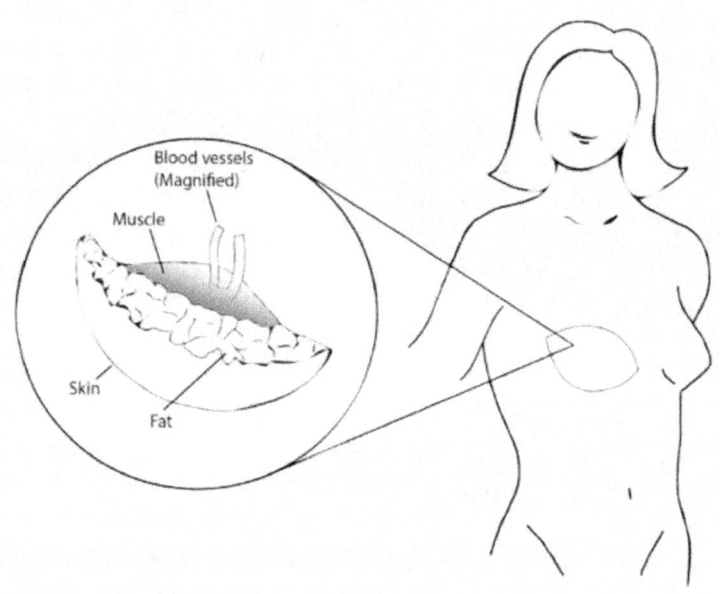

## Tissue Used To Rebuild Breast Shape

One of the typical areas where patients have fatty tissue available is in the lower abdomen, and often the patient has excess fat in this area. This is actually the first choice for tissue and it is known as the transverse rectus abdominis myocutaneous flap, which is better known as a TRAM flap. When a patient has excess fat in the lower abdominal area, below the navel, the flap and skin removal is similar to a tummy tuck, so we also achieve some body contouring in this area. A lot of our patients like that, because now they've gotten rid of their tummy that they didn't like.

In a typical TRAM flap, the incision and closure for the abdomen is down at the lower part of the abdomen, which is relatively hidden underneath underwear or a bathing suit. There are scars and they do go from hip to hip, but they're very well hidden in most patients. It's the same incision as a tummy tuck and pretty much the same thing as a C-section scar.

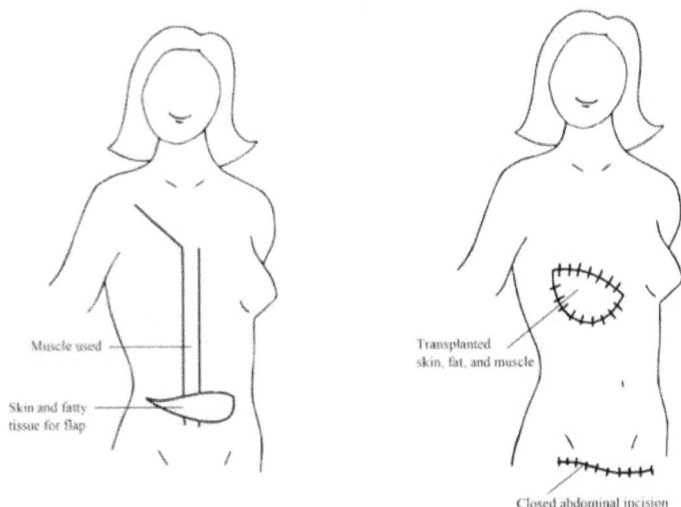

Muscle used

Skin and fatty
tissue for flap

Transplanted
skin, fat, and muscle

Closed abdominal incision

**TRAM Flap Incisions**

If the patient does not have enough fat and skin in the lower abdomen, we can use what is called a latissimus dorsi myocutaneous flap, or a LAT flap. In this case the tissue comes from the back.   Many times, the latissimus flap also requires an implant because the amount of fatty tissue that we can get from the back is somewhat limited, unlike the amount of fatty tissue that most of the time can be taken from the tummy.

When using the latissimus flap from the back, there is a scar on the back. Many women don't like that scar on their back, because if they are wearing a bathing suit, the scar will likely be visible.

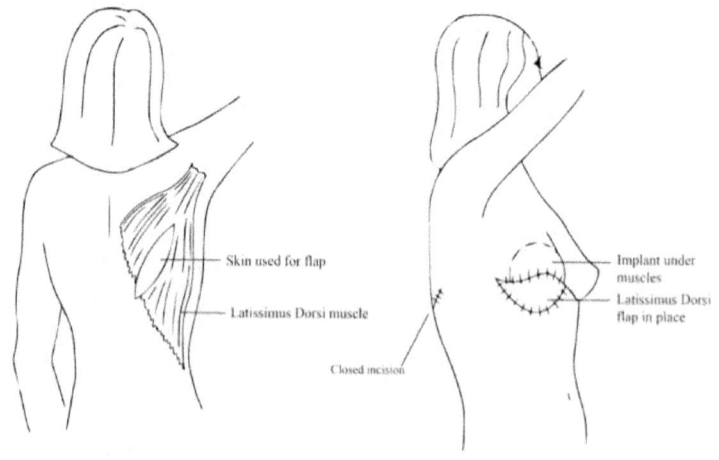

Skin used for flap

Latissimus Dorsi muscle

Closed incision

Implant under muscles

Latissimus Dorsi flap in place

## Latissimus Dorsi Flap

There is also the possibility of using the gluteal flap, which comes from the gluteal region or the buttock region of the patient. Those are the three most common flaps used, but the two main ones would be the TRAM flap and the latissimus flap.

In our patient consultations we help them understand the tradeoffs among the many reconstruction alternatives. One key choice as one can see relates to the use of a tissue expander and implants vs. using a tissue flap. If a patient doesn't have enough tissue from the tummy, that generally means they need the tissue expander followed by implant procedure. If they don't need irradiation and we can insert an expander at the same time as the mastectomy, the

28

patient will be left with only one linear scar in the breast where the general surgeon went through and removed the breast tissue.

When using a TRAM flap, we end up with more of an elliptical scar so the patient has extra incisions in and around the breast itself. There are many tradeoffs for the patient, so it is important to take all of these points into consideration when deciding on the specific procedures to be used.

*How do you reconstruct the nipple and areola? Are those done at the same time as the other procedures or at a later time?*

Nipples are reconstructed towards the end of the reconstructive process. I use small flaps of tissue to reconstruct the nipple using the patient's skin. Then about three months after the nipple reconstruction, we give it and the areola coloring by tattooing.

*How well will the reconstructed breast match the other breast?*

It can match quite nicely depending on the body habitus or physique of the patient. In a person who has a normal, straightforward body habitus where they're proportionate, they can have a pretty reasonable match between the two. If we are reconstructing both sides, both breasts are going to be symmetrical for the most part. Matching a reconstructed breast with a natural breast depends on the expertise of the surgeon and the tissue that we are working with.

Women want their breasts to match as much as possible and there are some limitations on matching. That is something that needs to be discussed with the surgeon. Many women choose to have the mastectomy performed on both sides so that they will have breasts that are very similar. The added benefit with removal of the opposite breast is that the chance of getting cancer in that breast will decrease very significantly.

That's a personal decision with the patient. There are some patients that still want to maintain the opposite breast; they don't want to operate on it. Breast reconstruction is custom work; it's unique for each patient and has to be tailored to each individual patient's wants and needs.

*How will a reconstructed breast feel to the touch?*

A reconstructed breast that has a silicone implant is going to have a soft feel, very similar to the other side. The saline implant breast is going to feel firmer and have a harder feel to it, less soft and it doesn't feel as natural. With a reconstruction using a tissue flap, the breast tends to feel like a normal breast because the soft subcutaneous fat that's used is going to feel soft like the opposite breast, because basically it's fatty tissue and most of the breast is fatty tissue. The silicone implants can approach that natural feel, depending on how much tissue is left from the mastectomy.

*Will there be any feeling in the reconstructed breast?*

The reconstructed breast has markedly decreased sensation. Studies have shown and patients report that over time, some of the nerves do grow back into the area, maybe over a period of about 18 months. The nipple is gone, so the nipple-areolar sensation is gone. When we do the nipple reconstruction, that nipple doesn't have sensation because the nerves to the nipple have been cut to remove the breast, so there is a significant loss of sensation to the breast. That's one reason that many women don't want to have a mastectomy on the other side; they want to preserve the nipple-areolar sensation on the opposite side.

*Is the mastectomy performed in a hospital surgical room?*

Although the procedure can be performed in an outpatient surgical center, most are performed in a hospital.

*Where is the reconstruction procedure performed?*

It can be done in a hospital or an outpatient surgical center, depending on the procedure. If we are using tissue expanders it can be done in an outpatient center or a hospital. When we use the flap procedures, the patient will typically need to stay in the hospital between two and three days because there is more recovery time for the patient. So with these procedures, we perform the surgery in a hospital.

*The reconstruction process has multiple phases, so how long a period of time is required to complete the reconstruction?*

That really depends on the patient and the specific procedures used. Since one of the more typical procedures is to use tissue expanders during the mastectomy and then later insert implants, we will use this case as an example. We will also assume the patient is having bilateral mastectomies, the pathology for the lymph nodes is negative during the surgery and the patient does not require chemotherapy or irradiation. This is a standard reconstruction.

Immediately following the mastectomies, we insert the tissue expanders and then allow time for the patient to recover. At three weeks, we start expanding that tissue, so it starts gradually expanding. It takes about two-and-a-half months or so to expand that tissue to get the appropriate breast size, but the time depends on the size of breasts the patient desires.

It's usually at about three to four months after the initial mastectomy and insertion of the tissue expanders that we will go back to surgery, take out the expander, and then put in the permanent breast implant. The implant would be either silicone or saline, depending on what the patient and the surgeon decided to do. The tissue is closed up, the patient recovers for a while, and then the nipple reconstruction is done about three months after that because we need to let the skin and the incision lines heal. Three months after the nipple reconstruction, we would tattoo the nipple.

*What is the recovery like for the patient having a breast reconstruction?*

Just as there are variables with the procedures used, the recovery will differ depending on the procedure. A patient having the reconstruction performed with tissue expander and implant will probably need a week or two off of work because they will be sore. This will depend on the physical activity and effort required for the job. In general, a patient with a tissue expander procedure can recover more quickly than somebody who's had the TRAM flap procedure. The TRAM flap recovery time is about six to eight weeks. With the tissue expander, though, the patient needs to come back to the office every week and have the tissue expanded until the proper size is achieved.

For driving, the patient cannot be taking narcotic drugs and has to feel comfortable that she can brake the car and steer the car. For the tissue expander route, I'd say that after about a week the patient should be able to be driving safely. With the flap, it's more likely to be two to three weeks in terms of being able to get out and drive a car and feel comfortable.

The patient will have pain and discomfort after surgery with any of these procedures, and we have a new device called a pain pump to handle initial pain management. The pain pump has a catheter that is placed underneath the operative site, usually on top of the muscles that allow numbing medicine to be essentially dripped onto the muscles. It comes from a reservoir and that reservoir allows this pain medicine to infiltrate to the tissues to help with postoperative pain. They work very nicely and they last about three to four days.

*Do the breast reconstructions interfere with any chemotherapy or radiation therapy treatment being provided to the patient?*

I like to have any chemotherapy and radiation therapy completed before we do the reconstruction. Some of the chemotherapy agents can actually delay wound healing, so my recommendation is to get any chemotherapy or radiation completed first. I personally like to wait about six months after irradiation to allow the body and the skin to heal because the irradiation does cause some damage to the skin. The skin can look somewhat like it's had a sunburn, so we can't operate on that tissue. It's not a really good idea to try to combine reconstructive surgery and chemotherapy at the same time, so for me, I like to have at least until six weeks after the chemotherapy is completed.

*How does aging affect the reconstructed breast?*

Breasts reconstructed with a flap procedure tend to mirror, somewhat, the natural aging process, whereas breasts with implants have less of a chance to show the natural aging process. As the aging process happens, the natural breast will sag, so after a number of years we may need to have the patient return and do a lifting procedure on the natural breast to achieve the best match at that time.

*Are there any specific risks or complications of breast reconstruction compared to other surgery?*

Every surgery has certain inherent risk to it, the usual things like bleeding, infection and the possibility of blood clots. Breast reconstruction has a slightly elevated risk of infection and that would need to be treated with antibiotics. Asymmetry can result and there may be a need for further surgery to further refine the appearance that the patient and the doctor want. As mentioned preciously the implant can fail at some point.

It should be obvious that a patient that has had cancer should not be smoking. Smoking affects the ability of tissue to heal and a patient with a tissue flap surgery could end up with the tissue dying.

*When a woman is seeking a plastic surgeon to discuss breast reconstruction, what specific qualifications of a plastic surgeon should she be looking for?*

Patients should seek out a plastic surgeon that is that is board certified by the American Board of Plastic Surgery. That's like a "seal of approval" from the major national certification board. Breast reconstruction is a specialized field within plastic surgery and it is important to be able to see the kind of work the plastic surgeon has done in terms of reconstruction, so patients will want to view their portfolio of before-and-after photos to demonstrate the results they have achieved. Years of experience and the quality of medical school and other training are other important indicators. The surgeon will need to be able to work in hospitals, so patients are advised to check the surgeon's hospital privileges.

*Where can I see examples of actual breast reconstruction patient results?*

My practice website has a number of before-and-after comparison photos. These can be viewed by visiting

http://www.BenChildersMD.com/galleries/breast-reconstruction

*Is breast reconstruction after mastectomy typically covered by insurance?*

In California, state law mandates that insurance covers both the reconstruction of the breast that's got cancer and then they cover the contralateral breast to match it, so there shouldn't really be an issue with reconstruction surgery.

# About The Author

Ben J. Childers, M.D., F.A.C.S. is a Board Certified Plastic Surgeon, a Fellow of the American College of Surgeons, and a member of the American Society of Plastic Surgeons. He practices at and is the owner of Riverside Plastic Surgery Associates, Inc. in Riverside, California. He also owns Sheer Beauty Medical Skin Care boutiques in Upland and Redlands, California.

Dr. Childers earned his BA degree in Chemistry from Eastern Kentucky University, graduating Cum Laude. He received his Medical Degree at the University of Louisville Medical School and competed his internship in General Surgery at Beth Israel Hospital Harvard Medical School. He completed his residency in General Surgery at Beth Israel Harvard Medical School and his residency in Plastic Surgery at Loma Linda University. Dr. Childers also completed a fellowship in Hand and Microsurgery at Beth Israel Deaconess Medical Center at Harvard Medical School.

With twenty of experience, 25,000 procedures and eight years of rigorous training at Harvard Medical School and Loma Linda University, he provides patients both experience and integrity.

Dr. Childers was named as one of the Top 10 Aesthetic Doctors in the United States and also as one of the Top 10 Plastic Surgeons in the West for 2014 -2015 by Aesthetic Everything® and Beautywire Magazine. Additional information can be seen by visiting:

https://madmimi.com/s/71c9b6

Dr. Childers offers full service cosmetic and reconstructive plastic surgery procedures. Standard cosmetic procedures offered include abdominoplasty (tummy tuck), liposuction, mastopexy (breast lift), breast augmentation and facial rejuvenation procedures such as facelift, blepharoplasty, and forehead lift. Areas of special interest to Dr. Childers are performing total body contouring surgery on patients after massive weight loss and breast reconstruction after mastectomy. Being able to restore form and function is one of the greatest rewards for a plastic surgeon.

A full range of non-invasive skin care procedures and products are found at his medical skin care boutiques. For those who are seeking non-surgical cosmetic solutions, medi-spa treatments are performed by certified aestheticians at the office in Riverside, and the Sheer Beauty Medical Skin Care boutiques in Upland and Redlands. Microdermabrasion, micro peels, Hydra facial, chemical peels, laser hair removal, IPL treatments, Fraxel Laser treatments, Botox, Thermage, and a full range of dermal anti-aging fillers are available.

For more information about Dr. Childers or to schedule a consultation, visit:

http://www.BenChildersMD.com

or call 951-781-4339

Riverside Plastic Surgery Associates, Inc. is located at

4605 Brockton Avenue, Suite 200
Riverside, CA 92506

For more information about Sheer Beauty Medical Skin Care, visit:

http://www.SheerBeautySkinCare.com.

Sheer Beauty Medical Skin Care is located in Upland and Redlands at

1875 North Campus Avenue, Suite B
Upland, CA 91784
909-985-5225

1615 West Lugonia Avenue
Redlands, CA 92374
909-798-4445

## Honors and Awards

The Joel Elkes Physicians and the Arts Award - 1989

The Harris Yett, M.D Orthopedic Award - 1990
Outstanding Orthopedic Resident of the Year
Beth Israel Hospital, Boston

First Place Poster Presentation - 1995
"HBO and Necrotizing Fasciitis"
Annual Post- Graduate Convention Alumni
Association
Loma Linda University Medical School

First Place: Best Resident Paper - 1995
Necrotizing Fasciitis- 122 Consecutive Cases
Tri-County Surgical Society 38th Annual Meeting
San Bernardino, CA

First Place Poster Presentation – 1999
Necrotizing Fasciitis-163 Consecutive Cases
Annual Post Graduate Convention LLUMC

Cambridge Who's Who Honored Member - 2010-2011
Registry of Executives and Professionals

National Institute of Medicine  - 2012
Distinguished Consultant

America's Top Surgeons - 2013-2014
Consumers' Research Council of America

Best Doctors Inland Empire Magazine - 2012-2015

Castle Connolly Top Doctor in Plastic Surgery - 2015

America's Top Breast Surgeons - 2014-2015
"The Top Plastic Surgeons in America Dedicated to Achieving Flawless Breast Surgery Results for the Most Discriminating Patients"

Top 10 Aesthetic Doctors in America and Top 10 Plastic Surgeons in The West
Aesthetic Everything® - 2014-2015

## Medical Publications

1. **Childers, B.J.,** Goldwyn, R.M., Ramos, D., Harris, J., The Long-term Results of Irradiation for Basal Cell Carcinoma of the Skin of the Nose. Plas. and Recon. Surg. Vol 93. No 6. May 1994.

2. **Childers, B.J.,** Hendricks, D.L., Tensor Fascia Lata Myocutaneous Free Tissue Transfer for Upper Abdominal Wall Defects. Plastic Surgical Forum. 63rd Annual Scientific Meeting Vol XVII 273-275. 1994.

3. **Childers, B.J.,** Hendricks, D.L., Tensor Fascia Lata Myocutaneous Free Tissue Transfer for   Upper Abdominal Wall Defects: A Report of Two Cases. American Society for Reconstructive Surgery Forum. 10th Anniversary  Meeting pages 201-202. 1994.

4. Nachreiner, R., **Childers, B.J.,** Hendricks, D.L., Rogers, F., Hardesty, R.A., : Necrotizing Fasciitis 122 Consecutive Cases.   Annual Meeting of the Southern California Chapter of the American College of Surgeons Forum. Page 99. 1995.

5. **Childers, B.J.,** Nachreiner, R., Hendricks, D.L., Rogers, F., and Hardesty, R.A., Necrotizing Fasciitis: A Retrospective Review of 122 Consecutive Cases. American College of Surgeons Surgical Forum Volume.  81st Clinical Congress of the American College of Surgeons. Volume XLVI pp 631-633. 1995.

6.  Nachreiner, R., **Childers, B.J.**, Kizziar, R., Hardesty, R.A. , Lo, T.: Adjuctive Hyperbaric Oxygen Therapy for Necrotizing Fasciitis: A Ten Year Experience. Plastic Surgical Forum 64th Annual Scientific Meeting Vol. XVIII pp 334-336. 1995.

7.  Hendricks, D.L. **Childers, B.J.**, Kachenmeister, R.: The Supercharged Osteocutaneous Free Fibula Flap: Extending the Osteocutaneous Fibula Flap to New Dimensions. Plastic Surgical Forum 64th Annual Scientific Meeting Vol XVIII pp 249-251. 1995.

8.  **Childers, B.J.**, Rohrer, P., Hardesty, R.A., An Anatomic Review and Transaxillary Endoscopic Augmentation Mammaplasty. Plastic Surgical Forum 64th Annual Scientific Meeting Vol XVIII pp 189-191. 1995.

9.  **Childers, B.J.**, Hendricks, D.L. Nasolabial Fasciocutaneous Free Flap for Facial Defects. Journal of Reconstructive Microsurgery October Vol 13 #7. 1997, pp 515-518.

10. Oberg, K.C., Robles, A.E., Ducsay, C.A., Rasi, C.R., Rouse, G.A., **Childers, B.J.**, Evans M.L., Kirsch, W.M., Hardesty, R.A.: Endoscopic Intrauterine Surgery in Primates Overcoming Technical Obstacles. Surgical Endoscopy In Press.

11. Oberg, K.C., Robles, A.E., Ducsay C.A., **Childers, B.J.** Gates D.L., Kirsch W.M., Hardesty, R.A., Endoscopic Creation of and Repair of Cleft Lip-Like Defects in Fetal Lambs. Min Invas Ther 4 (suppl #1): 57 (P-47). 1995.

12. Shusterman, M., Williams, S.R. **Childers, B.J.**, Soft Tissue Injection of Hydrocarbons: A Case Report and Review of the Literature. Journal of Emergency Medicine, Vol. 17 No.1, pp 63-65, 1999.

13. Oberg, K.C., Robles, A.E., Ducsay, C., **Childers, B.J.**, Rasi, C.R., Gates, D.L., Kirsch, W.M., Hardesty, R.A., Endoscopic Excision and Repair of Simulated Bilateral Cleft Lips in Fetal Lambs. Plas and Reconstr Surgery Vol 102. No 1. July 1998.

14. **Childers, B.J.**, Potyondy, L.D., Nachreiner, R., Rogers, F., Childers, E., Oberg, K.C., Hendricks, D.L., Hardesty, R.A., The Flesh Eating Disease "Necrotizing Fasciitis: A Fourteen-Year Retrospective Study of 163 Consecutive Cases" The American Surgeon, Vol. 68 Feb, 2002 pp 109-116.

15. **Childers, B.J.**, Andreasen, T., Green, S., AlloDerm Acellular Dermal Graft in the Treatment of Purpura Fulminans. Proceedings of the American Burn Association Journal of Burn Care and Rehabilitation Jan/Feb 2000 Volume 21 Number1, Part 2 Page S223.

16. **Childers, B.J.,** Andreasen, T., Green, S., AlloDermAcellular Dermal Graft in the Treatment of Purpura Fulminans. Plastic Surgical Forum 69th Annual Scientific Meeting September 2000.

17. Andreasen, T., Green, S., **Childers, B.J.,** Massive Infectious Soft Tissue Injury: Diagnosis and Management of Necrotizing Fasciitis and Purpura Fulminans. Plastic and Reconstructive Surgery, April 1,2001 Vol. 107, No 4.

18. Lamberton, G.R., Pereau, M., Illes, K., **Childers, B.J.,** Oberg, K.C., Szalay, A.A.: Generation and Characterization of bioluminescent *Streptococcus pyogenes*. Accepted for Publication in Luminescence. In press.

19. **Childers, B.J.** , Cobanov, Brando., Acute Infectious Purpura Fulminans: A 15-Year Retrospective Review of 28 Consecutive Cases. American Surgeon, January 2003. Vol. 69 pp 86-90.

**Textbook Chapters**

1. Upton, J., **Childers, B.J.,** Omental Free Flap In Russel-Zamboni: Microvascular      Free Flaps. In press 1997.

2. Upton, J., **Childers, B.J.,** Congenital Hand Surgery In Weinzweig, J.: Plastic  Surgical Secrets In press 1997, 2010.

## Presentations

1. **Childers, B.J.,** Hendricks, D.L.: Tensor Fascia Lata Myocutaneous Free Tissue Transfer for Upper Abdominal Wall Defects. Poster presentation ASPRS 63rd Annual Scientific Meeting. October 1994.

2. **Childers, B.J.,** Infection Fact or Fiction- Lecture at the 4th Annual Integrated Wound Symposium Veterans Administration Hospital Loma Linda. Ontario, CA. October 1994.

3. **Childers, B.J.,** Treatment Modalities for Difficult Wounds. Lecture at the 4th Annual Integrated Wound Symposium Veterans Administration Hospital Loma Linda. Ontario, CA. October 1994.

4. **Childers, B.J.,** Hendricks, D.L., Tensor Fascia Lata Myocutaneous Free Tissue Transfer for Upper Abdominal Wall Defects. Research Day at the Pettis V.A. Hospital Loma Linda, CA. November 1994.

5. Rohrer, P., **Childers, B.J.,** Hardesty, R.A., Endoscopic Breast Implants: A Clinical and Anatomic Presentation. Newport Beach, CA. October 1994.

6.  **Childers, B.J.,** Hendricks, D.L. Tensor Fascia Lata Myocutaneous Free Tissue Transfer for Upper Abdominal Wall Defects: A Report of Two Cases. Poster Presentation at the American Society for Reconstructive Microsurgery Tenth Anniversary Meeting. January 12-14, 1995.

7.  **Childers, B.J.,** Lecture: Necrotizing Fasciitis. Inland Empire Association of Enterostomal Theraists. Loma Linda, CA. January 19, 1995.

8.  Nachreiner, R., **Childers, B.J.,** Hendricks, D.L., Rogers, F., Hardesty, R.A., Necrotizing Fasciitis: 122 Consecutive Cases. Annual Meeting of the Southern California Chapter of the American College of Surgeons. Indian Wells, CA. January 20-22, 1995.

9.  **Childers, B.J.,** Hendricks, D.L., Tensor Fascia Lata Myocutaneous Free Tissue Transfer for Upper Abdominal Wall Defects. Poster Presentation at the Annual Post Graduate Convention Alumni Association of the School of Medicine. Loma Linda, CA. March 5-8, 1995.

10. **Childers, B.J.,** Rohrer, P., Hardesty, R.A., Advances in Plastic Surgery: Poster Presentation at the Annual Post Graduate Convention Alumni Association of the School of Medicine Loma Linda University. Loma Linda, CA March 5-8, 1995.

11.   Nachreiner, R., **Childers, B.J.**, Kizzar, R., Hardesty, R.A., Lo, T., HBO and Necrotizing Fasciitis Poster Presentation at the Annual Post Graduate Convention Alumni Association of the School of Medicine Loma Linda University. Loma Linda, CA. March 5-8, 1995.

12.   Hardesty, R.A., Oberg, K., **Childers, B.J.**, Robles, A., Endoscopic Intrauterine Cleft Lip Repair. Perspectives and Advances in Plastic Surgery Symposium. Olympic Valley, CA. Feb 20-25, 1995.

13.   Lo, T., Nachreiner, R., **Childers, B.J.**, Kizzlar, R., Hyperbaric Oxygen Therapy as an Adjunctive Therapy for Necrotizing Fasciitis. Winter Symposium on Baromedicine. Steamboat Springs, Colorado., January 20, 1995.

14.   **Childers, B.J.**, Nachreiner, R., Hendricks, D.L., Rogers, F., Hardesty, R.A., Necrotizing Fasciitis: A retrospective Review of 122 Consecutive Cases. Tri-County Surgical Society 38th Annual Meeting. San Bernardino, CA. May 18, 1995.

15.   **Childers, B.J.**, Webster, J., Hendricks, D.L., Two Stage Treatment of a Broncho-Pleural-Cutaneous Fistula with Pectoralis Major Muscle Flap. Tri-County Surgical Society 38th Annual Meeting. San Bernardino, CA. May 18, 1995.

16. Vanderlindin, S., **Childers, B.J.**, Hendricks, D.L., Use of Spare Parts to Reconstruct Tumor Ablation Defects of the Chest Wall. Tri-County Surgical Society 38th Annual Meeting. San Bernardino, CA. May 18, 1995.

17. **Childers, B.J.**, Hendricks, D.L., Nasolabial Fasciocutaneous Free Tissue Transfer for Cheek Defects. 45th Annual Meeting of the California Society of Plastic Surgeons, INC. May 25-29, 1995 Napa, California.

18. **Childers, B.J.**, Nachreiner, R., Hendricks, D.L., Rogers, F., Hardesty, R.A., Necrotizing Fasciitis: 122 Consecutive Cases. 45th Annual Meeting of the California Society of Plastic Surgeons, INC. May 25-29, 1995 Napa, CA.

19. Hardesty, R.A., Oberg, K., **Childers, B.J.**: Intruterine Fetal Surgery: Past Present and Future. University of Pittsburgh, Division of Plastic and Reconstructive Surgery. May 10, 1995, Pittsburgh, PA.

20. Oberg, K., Robles, A., Ducsay, C., **Childers, B.J.**, Gates, D., Kirsch, W., Hardesty, R.A., Endoscopic Creation of Cleft Lip-Like Defects in Fetal Lambs. Society for Minimally Invasive Therapy. September 21-24, 1995. Portland, Oregon.

21. **Childers, B.J.**, Nachreiner, R., Hendricks, D.L., Rogers, F., Hardesty, R.A., Necrotizing Fasciitis: A Retrospective Review of 122 Consecutive Cases. American College of Surgeons Surgical Forum Volume. 81st Clinical Congress of the American College of Surgeons. New Orleans, LA. October 22-27, 1995.

22. **Childers, B.J.**, Rohrer, P., Hardesty, R.A., An Anatomic Review and Transaxillary Endoscopic Augmentation Mammaplasty. ASPRS Forum October 1995.

23. Nachreiner, R., **Childers, B.J.**, Kizzlar, R., Hardesty, R.A., Lo, T., Adjunctive Hyperbaric Oxygen therapy for Necrotizing Fasciitis: A Ten Year Experience. ASPRS Forum October 1995.

24. **Childers, B.J.**, Hendricks, D.L., Kachenmeister, R., The Supercharged Osteocutaneous Free Fibula Flap: Extending the Osteocutaneous Fibula Flap to New Dimensions. ASPRS Forum October 1995.

25. **Childers, B.J.** Necrotizing Fasciitis. Grand Rounds Loma Linda University Department of Surgery. December 6, 1995.

26. Vanderlindin, S., **Childers, B.J.**, Yu, L., Hendricks, D.L., Use of Spare Parts to Reconstruct Tumor Ablation Defects of the Chest Wall. American Association For Hand Surgery Annual Meeting. January 10-13, 1996, Palm Springs, CA.

27. **Childers, B.J.,** Hendricks, D.L. The Nasolabial Fasciocutaneous Free Flap for Cheek Defects. "A Case Report". American Society for Reconstructive Microsurgery Annual Meeting. January 14-17, 1996. Tucson, Arizona.

28. Vanderlindin, S., **Childers, B.J.,** Yu.L., Hendricks, D.L., Use of Spare Parts to Reconstruct Tumor Ablation Defects of the Chest Wall. American Society for Reconstructive Microsurgery Annual Meeting. January 14-17, 1996. Tucson, Arizona.

29. Chang, P., Place, M., **Childers, B.J.,** Kim, P., Smith, D., Hendricks, D.L.,: The Extended Osteocutaneous Fibular Flap: An Anatomic Investigation . Annual Meeting of the Southern California Chapter American College of Surgeons. Santa Barbara, California Jan 19-21,1996.

30. Olberg, K.C., Robles, A., Ducsay, C.A., **Childers, B.J.,** Gates, D.L., Kirsch, W.M. & Hardesty, R.A. Endoscopic Creation and Cleft Lip-Like Defects in Fetal Lambs American Cleft Palate-Craniofacial Association. San Diego, California, April 22-27, 1996.

31. **Childers, B.J.,** Nachreiner, R., Rogers, F., Hendricks, D.L., Hardesty, R.A., Necrotizing Fasciitis: A Retrospective Review of 122 Consecutive Cases. Senior Residents Conference Dallas, Texas April 10-14, 1996.

32. **Childers, B.J.,** Grand Rounds Redlands Community Hospital. Management of Necrotizing Fasciitis. Redlands, California. April 15, 1996.

33. Hendricks, D.L., Kaidi, A., **Childers, B.J.:** Early Reconstruction of Gunshot Wounds to the Lower Face: A Treatment Algorithm for Successful Outcome. Tri-County Surgical Society 39th Annual Meeting. May 21, 1996.

34. Hendricks, D.L. Kaidi, A. **Childers, B.J.,** Immediate Definitive Reconstruction of Gunshot Wounds to the Face. California Society of Plastic Surgeons Annual Meeting. May 23-27, 1996.

35. **Childers, B.J.,** Webster, J., Hendricks, D.L., Treatment of Bronchocutaneous Pleural Fistula with Pectoralis Major Muscle Flap. California Society of Plastic Surgeons Annual Meeting. May 23-27, 1996.

36. Oberg, K.C., Robles, A.E., Ducsay, C., **Childers, B.J.,** Gates, D, Rasi, C., Chase, D., Kirsh, W.M. and Hardesty, R.A. Endoscopic Creation of Cleft-Lip-Like Defects in Fetal Lambs. Plastic Surgery Research Council Annual Meeting St. Louis, Missouri. June 7-10, 1996.

37. Upton, J., Mundlos, S., **Childers, B.J.,** Tattlebaum, A., Muragaki, Y., Olsen, B., The Genetic Sequence, Anatomical Variations, and Treatment of Central Polysyndactyly. Presented at the 24th Annual Meeting of the New England Hand Society, Dec 6, 1996, Sturbridge, MA.

38. Upton, J., Mundlos, S., **Childers, B.J.,** Tattlebaum, A., Muragaki, Y., Olsen, B., Genetics and Polydactyly. Presented to the New York Hand Society December 16, 1996.

39. **Childers, B.J.** Necrotizing Fasciitis. Visiting Professor Oregon Health Sciences Center Portland, Oregon Dec 12, 1996.

40. Oberg, K.C., Robles, A., Ducsay, C., **Childers, B.,** Evans, M., Rasi, C., Kirsh, W.M., Hardesty, R.A., Endoscopic Intrauterine Surgery in Primates: Overcoming Technical Obstacles. Society of American Gastrointestinal Endoscopic Surgeons Scientific Session. March 21-22, 1997 San Diego, CA.

41. A retrospective Review of 55 Consecutive Adult and Children Reconstructions **Childers, B.J.,** Upton, J., Wolfort, F., Free Flap Reconstruction for Oropharyngeal. New England Society of Plastic and Reconstructive Surgeons. May 30-June 1, 1997.

42. **Childers, B.J.,** Oropharyngeal Reconstruction: *The Patient, the Surgeon, the Flap(s),* University of California, San Diego. Department of Surgery Grand Round Presentation Sept 6, 1997.

43. **Childers, B.J.,** Ferraro, N., Wolfort, F., Upton, J. Free Flap Reconstruction for Oropharyngeal Defects: A Retrospective Review of 55 Consecutive Adult and Children Reconstructions, Plastic Surgery Research Council Annual Meeting, April 4-7, 1998.

44. Eichenber, B., Hendricks, D.L., **Childers, B.J.,** Alterations in the Anticoagulant Pathway Manifesting as Failed Microvascular Reconstruction. Plastic Surgery Research Council Annual Meeting April 4-7, 1998.

45. **Childers, B.J.,** Cohen, A., Rogers, F., Free Soft Tissue Pollicization to Salvage a Completely Degloved Thumb. American Association for Hand Surgery. 1998 Annual Meeting, Jan 13-16, 1999. Poster.

46. **Childers, B.J.,** Potyondy, L.D., Nachreiner, R., Rogers, F., Childers, E., Oberg, K.C., Hendricks, D.L., Hardesty, R.A., The Flesh Eating Disease "Necrotizing Fasciitis: A Fourteen-Year Retrospective Study of 163 Consecutive Cases" Annual Meeting of the Southern California Chapter of the American College of Surgeons. Santa Barbara, CA. January 22-24, 1999.

47.  Eichenberg, B., Sills, S., Wongworwat, A., **Childers, B.,** Hendricks, D.L., Hypercoaguable States in Microsurgery. Annual Meeting of the Southern California Chapter of the American College of Surgeons. Santa Barbara, CA. January 22-24, 1999.

48.  **Childers, B.J.,** Cohen, A., Rogers, F., Free Soft Tissue Pollicization to Salvage a Completely Degloved Thumb Annual Meeting of the Southern California Chapter of the American College of Surgeons. Santa Barbara, CA. January 22-24, 1999.

49.  Hazani, R., Kaidi, A., **Childers, B.J.,** Ciletti, S., Hardesty, R.A., Rogers, F., Johnson, C., Surreptitious Injection of Mineral Oil: A Case Presentation of Sclerosing Lipogranulomatosis. Presented at 49th Annual Meeting California Society of Plastic Surgeons May 27-31, 1999.

50.  Cohen, A., **Childers, B.J.:** Fibrous Dysplasia of the Sternum. Presented at 49th Annual Meeting California Society of Plastic Surgeons May 27-31, 1999.

51.  **Childers, B.J.,** Potyondy, L.D., Nachreiner, R., Rogers, F., Childers, E., Oberg, K.C., Hendricks, D.L., Hardesty, R.A., The Flesh Eating Disease "Necrotizing Fasciitis: A Fourteen-Year Retrospective Study of 163 Consecutive Cases" Annual Meeting ASPRS New Orleans October 1999.

52. **Childers, B.J.,** Andreasen, T., Green, S., AlloDerm Acellular Dermal Graft in the Treatment of Purpura Fulminans. American Burn Association 32nd Annual Meeting March 14-17, 2000.

53. **Childers, B.J.,** Andreasen, T., Green, S., AlloDerm Acellular Dermal Graft in the Treatment of Purpura Fulminans. Annual Post Graduate Convention Loma Linda University March 4-6, 2000.

54. **Childers, B.J.,** Andreasen, T., Green, S., AlloDerm Acellular Dermal Graft in the Treatment of Purpura Fulminans. Annual Meeting American Society of Plastic Surgeons, September 2000.

55. **Childers, B.J.** Johnson, B.J. Plastic Surgery Coding Update. American Academy of Professional Coders Annual National Meeting, Las Vegas, Nevada. April 2001.

56. Kelly, I., Lamberton, G., Chrisler, J., **Childers, B.J.,** Oberg, K.,: Murine Model for Bruise and Hematoma Formation. Presented at Annual Scientific Meeting of the American College of Surgeons Southern California Chapter. Santa Barbara, California January 19-21, 2001.

57. Andreasen, T., Swenson, R., Yu, L., Hendricks, D.L., **Childers, B.J.,:** The Use of Spare Part Fillet Flaps for Reconstructing Tumor Ablation Defects and Traumatic Wounds Presented at Annual Scientific Meeting of the American College of Surgeons Southern California Chapter. Santa Barbara, California January 19-21, 2001.

58. Andreasen, T., Swenson, R., Yu, L., Hendricks, D.L., **Childers, B.J.,:** The Use of Spare Part Fillet Flaps for Reconstructing Tumor Ablation Defects and Traumatic Wounds Presented at Annual Scientific Meeting of the American Society of Plastic Surgeons. Orlando, Florida. October 2001.

59. **Childers, B.J.,** Cobanov, B., : Acute Infectious Purpura Fulminans: A 15 Year Retrospective Review of 28 Consecutive Cases. Presented at the Annual Scientific Meeting of the American College of Surgeons Southern California Chapter. Santa Barbara, California January 18-20, 2002.

60. **Childers, B.J.,** Doezie, A. Muscle Stapling technique for Muscular Musculocutaneous Junction Lacerations in the Upper Extremity Presented at the Annual Scientific Meeting of the American College of Surgeons Southern California Chapter. Santa Barbara, California January 18-20, 2002.

61. **Childers,** B.J., Kim Y., Use of Halo for Immobilization of Patients Undergoing Total Calvarial Reconstruction. Presented at Annual Scientific Meeting of Society of Plastic Surgeons. San Antonio, Texas October 2002.

62. **The Pink Ribbon Place Presents" Breast Cancer: Now What?"** Featured quest specialist. Community Center, 10540 Magnolia Ave, Riverside CA, November 4, 2009.

## International and Community Service

1.  Loma Linda University Medical Center
    Division of Plastic and Reconstructive
    Surgery Medical Outreach Program, Mexicali,
    Mexico. Volunteer Surgeon, November 1994.

2.  Loma Linda University Medical Center
    Division of Plastic and Reconstructive
    Surgery Medical Outreach Program,
    Montomorales, Mexico. Volunteer Surgeon.
    June 1995.

3.  Donation of Horses to New Girls and Women
    Center for Equine Therapy. September 2012.

4.  Supporter of Claremont Club, Claremont,
    California 2013, 2014 Cancer Outreach Charity.

5.  Sponsor of National BRA Day USA, American
    Society of Plastic Surgeons Plastic Surgery
    Educational Foundation, 2014, 2015.

## Hospital Affiliations

1. Riverside Community Hospital
2. Loma Linda University Medical Center
3. Loma Linda Children's Hospital
4. Loma Linda Community Hospital
5. San Antonio Community Hospital
6. Premier Out Patient Surgery Center
7. Glenwood Surgery Center